THE *Skinny*
PRESSURE COOKER
COOKBOOK

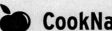 CookNation

THE SKINNY PRESSURE COOKER COOKBOOK

ISBN 978-1-909855-61-8

A CIP catalogue record of this book is available from the British Library

• •

DISCLAIMER

This book is designed to provide information on dishes that can be made in electric pressure cooker appliances; results may differ if alternative devices are used.
Some recipes may contain nuts or traces of nuts. Those suffering from any allergies associated with nuts should avoid any recipes containing nuts or nut based oils.

This information is provided and sold with the knowledge that the publisher and author do not offer any legal or other professional advice.

In the case of a need for any such expertise consult with the appropriate professional.

This book does not contain all information available on the subject, and other sources of recipes are available.

Every effort has been made to make this book as accurate as possible. However, there may be typographical and or content errors. Therefore, this book should serve only as a general guide and not as the ultimate source of subject information.

This book contains information that might be dated and is intended only to educate and entertain.

The author and publisher shall have no liability or responsibility to any person or entity regarding any loss or damage incurred, or alleged to have incurred, directly or indirectly, by the information contained in this book.

CONTENTS

MEAT   45

VEGETABLES   57

DESSERTS

INTRODUCTION

With our tasty pressure cooker recipes you will be cooking faster, healthier meals....the Skinny way.

The Pressure Cooker is an invaluable addition to the kitchen. Modern electric pressure cookers are safe, easy to use and perfect for cooking delicious & nutritious family meals in a fraction of the time traditional cooking methods require.

The Skinny Pressure Cooker Cookbook is a collection of carefully selected, fail-safe pressure cooker meals for the health conscious cook.

Every recipe falls below 300, 400 and 500 calories which means you can enjoy nutritious, delicious meals whilst still managing your weight.

With our tasty pressure cooker recipes you will be cooking faster, healthier meals....the Skinny way.

Cooking in an electric pressure cooker is an extremely efficient and healthy way to prepare food. Utilizing a wide variety of liquids such as water, vegetable, beef or chicken broth, low-fat gravies, fruit juice and healthy milk such as almond or soy can ensure a healthy meal in a short amount of time. Pressure-cooking times are much less than ordinary cooking and as the evaporation created is eliminated, only a small amount of liquid is required.

No matter what you are cooking, the liquids used must completely cover the bottom of the cooker so it will last during the entire cooking time. However, when it comes to cooking stews, soups and puddings, the amount of liquid needed is increased, but don't worry as all this has been taken into consideration in our recipes.

When it comes to cooking solid foods, a pressure cooker should never be more than two-thirds full as there must be enough room for the steam to circulate and do its job. Make sure there is enough space between the food and the lid to prevent the steam vent from getting blocked in any way. For liquids, the maximum amount should only be halfway from the base to allow for the liquids to boil.

You might have a favorite recipe that you would like to cook in your pressure cooker. If you have a recipe that is cooked traditionally in the oven, take one-third of the normal cooking time for cooking in your pressure cooker.

You might also like to invest in an immersion blender as it makes it so much easier to blend soup recipes into a creamy, smooth texture. It will save you time and energy. If you don't have one, then ladle the soup into a regular blender or food processor and blend slowly. Smaller batches can be done to minimize the risk of splashing.

You will notice that Himalayan sea salt is used in the recipes for seasoning. Himalayan sea salt is widely regarded as a healthier choice to regular sea salt. It is available at most health food markets and grocery stores in bulk for grinding fresh with each use. However feel free to use regular salt if you prefer.

These delicious recipes use simple and inexpensive fresh ingredients; are packed full of flavour and goodness, and show that you can enjoy maximum taste with minimum calories.

ABOUT COOKNATION

CookNation is the leading publisher of innovative and practical recipe books for the modern, health conscious cook. CookNation titles bring together delicious, easy and practical recipes making cooking for diets and healthy eating fast, simple and fun.

With a range of #1 best-selling titles - from the innovative 'Skinny' calorie-counted series, to the 5:2 Diet Recipes collection - CookNation recipe books prove that 'Diet' can still mean 'Delicious'!

Turn to the end of this book to browse all CookNation's recipe books.

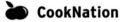 CookNation

Skinny
PRESSURE
COOKER SOUPS

SQUASH SOUP WITH CHICKEN AND APPLES

270 calories per serving

Ingredients

- 1 tablespoon of extra-virgin olive oil
- 1½ cup of chopped leaks or 8 green onions
- 2 cups of cooked chicken
- 4 cups of filtered water
- 4 Honey Crisp or Pink Lady apples – peeled and quartered
- 1 pound of butternut squash – peeled, seeded and chopped
- 1/3 cup of steel-cut oats
- 2 tablespoons of fresh ginger – minced or 1 teaspoon of ground ginger
- 1 tablespoon of curry powder
- 1 teaspoon Himalayan salt
- White Pepper to taste

Method

1 Heat the olive oil in the pressure cooker and add the leeks or green onions - sauté for at least one minute before adding the rest of the ingredients.

2 Lock the lid in place and bring the pressure to a high heat and cook for five minutes.

3 Turn OFF the heat and allow the pressure to come down naturally. It should take about 15 minutes.

4 Remove the lid and preferably use an immersion blender to puree the soup to a creamy, smooth texture or until any lumps are gone.

5 Season & serve.

CHEFS NOTE

Roast a bag of chopped walnuts in the oven at 375 degrees for about 10 minutes. It brings out their flavor and adds extra crunch to the soup.

SWAMP SOUP

SERVES 4

268 calories per serving

Ingredients

- 1 cup cooked chickpeas or garbanzo beans
- 4 fingerling potatoes – cut in half
- 3 cloves of garlic or 3 teaspoons of minced garlic from a jar
- 2 small yellow onions – peeled and quartered
- 1 bag of fresh, organic spinach
- Water or vegetable stock – enough to cover the vegetables in the pressure cooker
- 1 tbsp extra-virgin olive oil
- Himalayan sea salt and pepper to taste

Method

1 Place the chickpeas, potatoes, garlic cloves and onions in the pressure cooker. Add enough stock or water to cover them.

2 Lock the lid in place and bring it up to high pressure, then lower it and cook for about 10 minutes.

3 Allow the pressure to drop and remove the lid. Using an immersion blender, blend the soup until it is smooth and creamy.

4 Add the fresh spinach and olive oil. Lock the lid again and bring to a high pressure again. Lower the heat and let cook for about 2 minutes.

CHEFS NOTE

Many whole-food markets offer cooked chickpeas in their deli section or freezer section that are ready to use. If you must used canned chickpeas, make sure you rinse them first before adding them to your electric pressure cooker.

TOMATO BASIL SOUP

156 calories per serving

Ingredients

- 2 tablespoons of extra-virgin olive oil
- 1 red onion – chopped finely
- 8 Roma tomatoes – chopped
- 2 teaspoons of tomato paste
- Himalayan sea salt and pepper to taste
- 1 cup of chicken or vegetable broth
- ¾ cup of plain Almond milk
- 6 leaves of fresh basil - chopped

Method

1 Heat the olive oil in the bottom of the pressure cooker and cook the onions for about 5 minutes.

2 Add the tomatoes, tomato paste, salt, pepper and broth. Mix well. Lock the lid in place and bring the pressure up to high heat. Reduce it to low and maintain the pressure, cooking for 15 minutes.

3 Once the pressure has dropped, open the lid and add the almond milk and fresh basil.

4 Using an immersion blender, blend the soup until smooth and creamy.

CHEFS NOTE

Use fresh tomatoes or look for a box of Pomi tomatoes, they are convenient and delicious.

ITALIAN WEDDING SOUP

SERVES 4

220 calories per serving

Ingredients

- 2 tablespoons of extra-virgin olive oil
- ½ pound of ground turkey breast
- 1 small red onion – diced
- ½ cup pearl barley
- 3 garlic cloves or 3 teaspoons of minced garlic packed in olive oil
- 1 bag of fresh spinach
- 4 cups of chicken or vegetable broth
- ½ cup of mild salsa

Method

1 Pour 1 tablespoon of olive oil in the bottom of the pressure cooker. Add the turkey meats and cook. Spoon the meat out and set aside.

2 Add the other tablespoon of olive oil and cook the onions and garlic for about one minute. Add barley, the cooked turkey meat, lentils and then add enough chicken broth to cover the ingredients in the pressure cooker.

3 Lock the lid in place and bring the pressure to high. Then lower the heat and cook for 15 minutes.

4 Using the automatic release method on your pressure cooker, remove the lid and add the lentils, spinach, salsa and remaining broth. Heat thoroughly and serve.

CHEFS NOTE
You can also try adding some lentils if you like.

15

LENTIL-POTATO SOUP

260
calories per
serving

Ingredients

- 1 tablespoon of extra-virgin olive oil
- 1 red onion – chopped
- 1 small bag of carrot sticks
- 2 bay leaves
- 2 sprigs of fresh thyme – leaves removed or 1 teaspoon of dried thyme
- 1 teaspoon of ground savory
- 6 cups of chicken or vegetable broth
- 2 fingerling potatoes
- ½ cup of lentils
- Himalayan sea salt and pepper to taste

Method

1 Heat the olive oil in the pressure cooker over medium heat and sauté the chopped onions for about 2 minutes.

2 Add the carrots and cook for another minute. Add the bay leaves, thyme, savory, broth, potatoes and lentils. Stir well.

3 Lock the lid in place and bring the pressure up to high and the mixture boils. Reduce the heat and cook for about 12 minutes.

4 Remove the lid and discard the bay leaves and season with sea salt and pepper to taste.

CHEFS NOTE
Serve with a sprinkling of Parmesan cheese.

ROTISSERIE-CHICKEN VEGETABLE SOUP

320 calories per serving

Ingredients

- 1 tablespoon of extra-virgin olive oil
- 2 garlic cloves – minced
- 1 box of Pomi chopped tomatoes or 4 tomatoes – chopped
- 1 potato – cut into chunks
- 1 cup of carrot sticks
- 1 small yellow onion – chopped
- 2 celery sticks – chopped
- 8 ounces of sliced Portabella mushrooms
- 2 sprigs of fresh thyme – leaves only or 1 teaspoon of dried thyme

- 1 sprig of fresh rosemary – leaves only or 1 teaspoon of dried rosemary
- 2 bay leaves
- Himalayan sea salt and pepper to taste
- 2 cups of pulled Rotisserie-chicken breast
- 1 10-ounce package of frozen peas - thawed
- 1 10-ounce package of frozen corn – thawed
- ½ cup of fresh parsley – minced

Method

1 Heat the olive oil in the pressure cooker and sauté garlic for about 12 seconds. Add tomatoes, potatoes, carrots, onions, celery, mushrooms, thyme, rosemary, bay leaves and chicken - season with salt and pepper to taste. Lock the lid in place and bring to high pressure. Cook for 12 minutes maintaining pressure.

2 Once cooking is complete, reduce the pressure with the automatic release method. Stir in the peas, corn and parsley. Bring to a boil over medium heat and cook for about 5 minutes.

3 Check the seasoning & serve.

CHEFS NOTE

Try and source Portabella mushrooms if you can, they are tastier than regular white button mushrooms.

MEXICAN SOUP

SERVES 4

320 calories per serving

Ingredients

- 1 cup cooked Rotisserie chicken – pulled from the bone and shredded
- 1 bag of carrot sticks
- 3 celery sticks – chopped
- 1 red onion – chopped
- 7 ounces canned kidney beans – rinsed thoroughly and drained
- 1 box of Pomi tomatoes – chopped or 5

- fresh tomatoes – chopped
- 6 cups of chicken broth
- 1 10-ounce bag of frozen corn
- 1 teaspoon of ground cumin
- Himalayan sea salt and pepper to taste
- 3 garlic cloves – minced or 3 teaspoons of chopped garlic from a jar

Method

1 Place all ingredients in your pressure cooker and lock the lid in place. Bring to a boil at high pressure and cook for five minutes.

2 Release the pressure naturally and let cook for another 10 minutes.

3 Serve with a whole-grain tortilla chip as a garnish.

CHEFS NOTE
Add some plain tortilla chips to serve.

PUMPKIN SOUP WITH BLACK BEANS

210 calories per serving

Ingredients

- 1 tablespoon of extra-virgin olive oil
- 1 medium onion – diced
- 4 garlic cloves – minced or 4 teaspoons of minced garlic from a jar
- 1 heaping teaspoon of ground cumin
- 1 chipotle pepper – minced or 1 teaspoon of adobo sauce
- 2 cups of pumpkin – cubed

- 1 cup black beans – rinsed thoroughly and drained
- 3 Roma tomatoes – chopped
- 2 cups of vegetables stock
- Himalayan sea salt and pepper to taste
- ½ cup of cilantro – minced
- Juice of one lime

Method

1 Place all ingredients in your electric pressure cooker. Secure the lid and bring to a boil under high pressure. Reduce heat to medium and cook for 10 minutes. Release the pressure naturally or by using the automatic pressure release.

2 Using an immersion blender, blend the soup until smooth and creamy or you can leave it chunky.

3 Stir in the cilantro, lime juice and serve with a dollop of Greek plain yogurt or whole-grain tortilla chips.

CHEFS NOTE

Substitute acorn, butternut or winter squash for pumpkin if it's not available.

Skinny
PRESSURE
COOKER SEAFOOD

STEAMED LOBSTERS
SERVED WITH FRESH ASPARAGUS AND PORCINI
MUSHROOM RISOTTO ▶ SEE PAGE 23

495
calories per serving

Ingredients

- 1 bunch of fresh Asparagus – ends broken off
- 1 tablespoon of extra-virgin olive oil
- 1 teaspoon of garlic powder
- 1 cup of white wine or water

- 4 8-ounce lobster tails
- Himalayan sea salt and pepper
- Melted butter

Method

1 Preheat oven to 375 degrees. Spread asparagus out on a cookie sheet with a lip around the edges. Drizzle the olive oil over the top and sprinkle with garlic powder. Bake in the oven for 15 minutes.

2 Place the lobster tails inside the pressure cooker, shell side down. Pour wine over all. Secure the lid in place and bring up to high pressure. Cook for 3 minutes.

3 Release the pressure using the automatic pressure release. Remove the lid and season with sea salt.

4 Serve with melted butter on the side.

CHEFS NOTE
The lobsters will taste delicious whether they are cooked in wine or water.

MUSHROOM RISOTTO WITH PORCINI MUSHROOMS

Ingredients

- 8 cups of low-sodium chicken broth
- 1 ounce of dried porcini mushrooms
- 2 tablespoons olive oil
- 1 red onion - chopped
- 10 ounces of Portabella mushrooms - chopped
- 2 cloves of garlic - minced
- 1 cup of brown rice
- 2/3 cup of dry white wine
- Himalayan sea salt and pepper to taste

Method

1 In a medium saucepan, bring the broth to a boil. Add the porcini mushrooms and set aside until the mushrooms are tender, about 5 minutes. Keep the broth warm over a very low heat.

2 In a large saucepan on medium heat, add the olive oil and onions and sauté until tender, about 8 minutes. Add the Portabella mushrooms and garlic. Using a slotted spoon, transfer the porcini mushrooms to a cutting board and chop the mushrooms before adding to the saucepan.

3 Sauté until all the mushrooms are tender and the juices evaporate, about 5 minutes. Stir in the rice and let it brown for a few minutes. Add the wine and cook until the liquid is absorbed, stirring often, about 2 minutes.

4 Add 1 cup of hot broth; simmer over medium-low heat until the liquid is absorbed, stirring often, about 3 minutes. Continue to cook until the rice is just tender and the mixture is creamy, adding more broth by the ladleful. Stir often, about 30 minutes. The rice will absorb about 6 to 8 cups of broth.

5 Season with sea salt and pepper to taste.

BAKED TILAPIA WITH SHRIMP SAUCE

475 calories per serving

Ingredients

- 1 tbsp extra-virgin olive oil
- ¼ cup of whole-grain flour
- ½ cup of plain almond milk
- Himalayan sea salt and pepper
- Juice of one lemon
- 1 egg yolk
- 1 cup of cooked shrimp – chopped
- 1 cup of brown rice
- 1 head of broccoli – cut into pieces
- 4 4-ounce Tilapia filets

Method

1 Heat the olive oil in the bottom of the pressure cooker. Add the flour and milk and mix well. Cook until thickened.

2 Add the sea salt, pepper, egg yolk and cooked shrimp. Stir well.

3 Add the rice and broccoli and place tilapia filets on top of all. Season the filets with fresh ground pepper.

4 Secure the lid and bring up to high pressure. Cook for 8 minutes. Turn off and release the pressure naturally.

5 Season and serve.

CHEFS NOTE
Any fish will work for you if Tilapia filets are not available.

CITRUS TOPPED SALMON

375
calories per
serving

Ingredients

- 4 6-ounce salmon filets
- 1 teaspoon of onion powder
- Himalayan sea salt and pepper to taste
- 1 lemon – sliced
- 1 lime - sliced
- 1 orange – sliced
- 1 red onion – sliced
- 4 medium-size new red potatoes

- 1 16-ounce bag of fresh spinach
- 2 tablespoons of extra-virgin olive oil
- 2 tablespoons of sugar-in-the-raw
- 2 cups of fresh squeezed orange juice
- 2 tablespoons of cornstarch
- ¼ cup of soy sauce
- ¼ cup of apple cider vinegar

Method

1 Season the salmon filets with the onion powder, sea salt and pepper. Arrange the filets in the bottom of the pressure cooker. Top with fruit, onion slices, red potatoes and spinach.

2 Mix the olive oil, sugar, orange juice, cornstarch, soy sauce and vinegar in a bowl. Pour over all.

3 Secure the lid and bring up to high pressure. Cook for 10 minutes. Release the pressure with the automatic pressure release and keep warm for 5 minutes.

4 Serve immediately.

CHEFS NOTE

This recipe also work well with other fish filets however if they are particularly thin reduce the cooking time by a few minutes.

COD WITH FRESH ASPARAGUS AND SWEET POTATOES

397 calories per serving

Ingredients

- 4 6-ounce cod filets
- 1 bunch of fresh asparagus
- 2 large sweet potatoes – peeled and cut into small squares
- 2 tablespoons of fresh parsley – chopped
- 1 cup of white wine

- Juice of one lemon
- 2 garlic cloves – chopped
- 1 teaspoon of dried oregano
- 1 teaspoon of paprika

Method

1 Place the cod filets in the bottom of the pressure cooker and top with the fresh asparagus and sweet potatoes. Pour the wine and lemon juice over all. Season with sea salt and pepper – then sprinkle the garlic, oregano and paprika over all. Secure the lid and bring up to high pressure. Cook for 2 minutes.

2 Release the pressure using the automatic pressure release. Serve the cod immediately with asparagus.

3 Pour the wine and lemon juice liquid over all when serving.

CHEFS NOTE

One tablespoon of fresh oregano works well. For added flavor and crunch, sprinkle toasted almond slivers on top. Vegetable or chicken broth can be substituted for the wine.

STEAMED FISH FILLET WITH TOMATOES, OLIVES AND ANGEL HAIR

440
calories per serving

Ingredients

- ½ cup of water or white wine
- 8 ounces of angel hair pasta
- 4 6-ounce White fish filets
- 1 small container (8 ounces) of cherry tomatoes – sliced in half
- 1 cup of green or black olives
- 1 garlic clove – crushed
- 1 sprig of fresh thyme leaves or 1 teaspoon of dried thyme
- 1½ tablespoons of extra-virgin olive oil
- Himalayan sea salt and pepper to taste

Method

1 Pour the water or wine in the bottom of the pressure cooker. Place the angel hair pasta and filets in the water or wine and top with the tomatoes and olives.

2 Add the garlic, thyme and drizzle the olive oil over all - season with sea salt and pepper. Secure the lid and bring the pressure up to high. Cook for 5 minutes.

3 Release the pressure using the automatic pressure release. Open the lid and serve the filets immediately topped with tomatoes and olives.

CHEFS NOTE
The filets can be cooked at a lower pressure for 7-9 minutes, if you prefer. The pasta cooks in the liquid underneath the filets.

27

COCONUT-CURRY FILETS

487
calories per serving

Ingredients

- 4 6-ounce white fish filets
- ½ cup of lite coconut milk
- 1½ cups of white rice
- 2 cups of fresh or frozen peas
- 2 tablespoons of extra-virgin olive oil
- 2 Roma tomatoes – diced
- 1 red pepper – cut into strips
- 1 red onion – chopped

- 2 garlic cloves – minced
- 1 tablespoon of ground ginger
- 1 teaspoon of ground turmeric
- 2 tablespoons of ground cumin
- 1 teaspoon of hot red pepper flakes
- ½ teaspoon of fenugreek
- Himalayan sea salt to taste
- Juice of one lemon

Method

1 Place the fish in the coconut milk and set aside.

2 Heat the olive oil in the pressure cooker and cook the red peppers and onions. Add the spices, rice and peas.

3 Place the filets on top and pour the coconut milk over all. Add the tomatoes on top.

4 Secure the lid and bring the pressure up to high. Cook for 5 minutes.

5 Release the pressure using the automatic pressure release.

6 Serve immediately with the tomatoes, red peppers and onions on top.

7 Season with Sea salt and sprinkle lemon juice on top of each filet.

CHEFS NOTE
Frozen fish works well in this recipe. Of course, you can use 2 tablespoons of chopped fresh ginger instead of dried ginger in this recipe.

MEDITERRANEAN FILETS

495
calories per serving

Ingredients

- 4 6-ounce whitefish filets
- 1 small container of cherry tomatoes
- 8 fingerling potatoes – washed and dried
- 1 head of cauliflower – cut into pieces
- 2 sprigs of fresh thyme leaves or 1 teaspoon of ground thyme
- 1 cup of vegetable broth
- 2 tablespoons of pickled capers
- 1 cup of green olives
- 1 garlic clove – minced
- 2 tablespoons of extra-virgin olive oil
- Himalayan sea salt and pepper to taste
- More sprigs of thyme for garnish

Method

1 Place half of the cherry tomatoes, potatoes and cauliflower in the bottom of the pressure cooker. Add the fresh thyme and broth.

2 Place the filets on top. Sprinkle the capers, olives and garlic over the fish. Drizzle with olive oil and season with sea salt and pepper to taste.

3 Secure the lid and bring the pressure up to high. Cook for 5 minutes.

4 Reduce the pressure with the automatic pressure release.

5 Serve on individual plates and garnish with more cherry tomatoes and fresh thyme sprigs.

CHEFS NOTE

This recipe works well with salmon too.

SEAFOOD CHOWDER
WITH ROMAINE SALAD TOSSED IN PEANUT BUTTER VINAIGRETTE ▶ SEE PAGE 31

440 calories per serving

Ingredients

- 4 6-ounce haddock filets – cut into chunks
- 6 fingerling potatoes – cut into chunks
- 1 yellow onion – chopped
- 1 cup of plain almond milk
- ½ cup of chicken or vegetable broth
- ½ cup of plain Greek yogurt
- Himalayan sea salt and pepper to taste

Method

1 Place the fish chunks, potatoes, onion, almond milk, broth and water in the pressure cooker. Secure the lid and bring the pressure up to high. Cook for 10 minutes.

2 Release the pressure using the automatic pressure release. Open the lid and set the heat to medium low. Stir in the yogurt and season with sea salt and pepper to taste.

3 Continue to stir until the chowder is thickened.

4 Serve immediately.

CHEFS NOTE
Haddock is used in this recipe, however any white fish will work. For a healthier recipe, cream is replaced with plain Greek yogurt. It adds protein with less fat for a healthier chowder.

PEANUT BUTTER VINAIGRETTE

Ingredients

In a bowl, whisk together the following ingredients:
- ¼ cup of apple cider vinegar
- 1 tablespoon of fresh ground peanut butter
- ½ teaspoon of ground red pepper
- 1 teaspoon of Italian herbs
- 1 teaspoon of garlic powder
- ½ cup of extra virgin olive oil

Method

1 Place vinegar, peanut butter and spices in a bowl. Whisk in the olive oil until a smooth consistency forms.

2 Toss with Romaine lettuce, chopped tomato and sprinkle salad with 1 tablespoon of grated Parmesan.

GINGER ORANGE ROUGHY FILETS WITH SWEET POTATOES AND CARROTS

465 calories per serving

Ingredients

- 4 6-ounce Orange Roughy filets
- 2 large sweet potatoes – peeled and cut into squares
- 4 carrots – peeled and sliced
- 2 tablespoons of extra-virgin olive oil
- Juice of one orange
- Zest from one orange

- 2 tablespoons of fresh ginger – minced or 1 tablespoon of ground ginger
- 4 green onions – sliced 2-inches in length on the diagonal
- Himalayan sea salt and pepper to taste
- 1 cup of white wine

Method

1 Rub olive oil on both sides of the filets – season with sea salt and pepper to taste and set aside.

2 Place the sweet potatoes and carrots in the bottom of the pressure cooker. Add the filets on top. Mix together the orange juice, zest, ginger, green onions and wine. Pour over all.

3 Secure the lid and bring the pressure up to high. Cook for 7 minutes.

4 Release the pressure with the automatic pressure release. Serve immediately with juice from the bottom of the pressure cooker.

5 Garnish with fresh orange slices.

CHEFS NOTE
This recipe works well with a vegetable or side salad for a healthy meal.

Skinny
PRESSURE
COOKER POULTRY

BASIC ROASTED CHICKEN
WITH DIJON MUSTARD FINGERLING POTATOES AND CARROTS

495
calories per serving

Ingredients

- One whole chicken (3.5 pounds)
- Himalayan sea Salt and pepper
- 1 teaspoon of garlic powder
- 1 teaspoon of onion powder
- 1 teaspoon of ground thyme

- 2 tablespoons of extra-virgin olive oil
- 8 fingerling potatoes
- 4 carrots – peeled and sliced
- ¼ cup of Dijon mustard

Method

1 Liberally coat the chicken with all the spices. Heat the olive oil in the pressure cooker and brown the chicken on all sides.

2 Keep chicken in the pressure cooker. Mix the potatoes and carrots in mustard and pour on top of chicken.

3 Secure the lid and bring the pressure up to high. Allow 6 minutes per pound of chicken. Release the pressure by using the automatic pressure release method and remove the lid.

CHEFS NOTE

While the chicken is cooking in the pressure cook, use the time to chop up some of your favorite vegetables to roast in the oven. Cauliflower, carrots, sweet potatoes, beets and turnips work well. Drizzle with olive oil and your favorite seasonings for vegetables and roast in the oven for about 40 minutes at 375 degrees. The high heat caramelizes the vegetables for delicious flavor.

CLASSIC CHICKEN WITH BROWN RICE, CARROTS AND PEAS

492 calories per serving

Ingredients

- 4 6-ounce chicken breasts with the bone-in
- Himalayan sea salt and pepper to taste
- 1 tablespoon of extra-virgin olive oil
- 4 carrots – peeled and sliced
- 1 10-ounce package of frozen peas

- 1½ cups of brown rice
- 1 red onion – finely chopped
- 2 cups of low-sodium chicken broth or homemade broth
- 3 tablespoons of fresh parsley – minced
- Juice of one lemon

Method

1 Season chicken breasts with sea salt and pepper. Heat the oil in the pressure cooker pot and cook chicken breasts on both sides for about a minute on each side.

2 Add carrots, peas, rice, onions, a pinch of sea salt, rice and garlic. Secure the lid and bring up to high pressure. As soon as it reaches high pressure, reduce the heat to medium-low and cook for 15 minutes.

3 Release the pressure using the automatic release method and remove the lid. Transfer the chicken breasts to a serving platter and keep warm.

4 Sprinkle the remaining rice, peas and carrots with parsley and squeeze lemon juice over all.

5 Let stand for about 5 minutes. Fluff the rice with a fork and season with sea salt and pepper to taste. Serve the rice, peas and carrots with the chicken.

CHEFS NOTE

For a change from brown rice, you could also use quinoa (pronounced qeen-wa) for a healthy alternative.

CHICKEN MASALA

494
calories per serving

Ingredients

- 4 6-ounce boneless, skinless chicken breasts
- Himalayan sea salt and pepper to taste
- 1 tablespoon of extra-virgin olive oil
- 1 ½ cups of Portabella mushrooms – sliced
- ½ of a yellow onion – sliced

- 1 garlic clove – minced
- 2 tablespoons fresh basil – roughly chopped
- 1 tablespoon of dried Oregano
- 2 cups of Masala wine
- 1 box of noodles made from vegetables or rice (available in the pasta section)

Method

1 Season both sides of each chicken breast with sea salt and pepper. Heat the olive oil in the bottom of the pressure cooker and cook breasts about 1 minute on each side. Remove and set aside.

2 Add the mushrooms, onions, herbs and garlic. Cook for about 2 minutes stirring well. Turn off the heating element and add the wine.

3 Place the angel hair, broccoli and chicken breasts on top of everything and secure the lid. Bring the pressure cooker up to high pressure and cook for 15 minutes.

4 After the fifteen minutes, let the pressure drop naturally. It should take about 5 minutes. Unlock the lid. Place each chicken breast on a bed of angel hair, add some of the broccoli and pour a ladle-full of sauce over all. Enjoy!

CHEFS NOTE

If you prefer a thicker sauce, you can remove the chicken and mix together a tablespoon of potato starch and ¼ cup of water. Add this mixture to the wine sauce and heat through. Add the chicken back and coat them in the sauce – the longer they sit in the sauce, the thicker it gets.

CHICKEN PARMIGIANINO

499
calories per
serving

Ingredients

- ¼ cup whole-grain flour or rice flour
- ½ teaspoon of dried rosemary or 2 tablespoons of fresh rosemary – finely chopped
- ½ teaspoon dried basil or 2 tablespoons of fresh basil – finely chopped
- ½ teaspoon of garlic powder
- Himalayan sea salt and pepper to taste
- 4 6-ounce boneless, skinless chicken breasts – pounded evenly

- 1 ½ tablespoon of extra-virgin olive oil
- ½ cup of chicken broth – low sodium
- 1 garlic clove – chopped
- 1 jar of your favorite marinara or spaghetti sauce
- ½ cup red wine
- 6 ounces of spaghetti
- 1 head of broccoli – cut into small pieces
- Parmesan cheese for garnishing

Method

1 Combine the flour with all the spices and seasonings. Coat each chicken breast in the flour and set aside.

2 Heat the oil in the bottom of the pressure cooker and brown each chicken breast. You may cook 2 at a time. Remove.

3 Pour the broth, marinara sauce, garlic and wine into the pressure cooker. Mix well.

4 Add the spaghetti, broccoli and the chicken breasts in the sauce. Coat them well.

5 Lock the lid and bring to high pressure. Cook for 10 minutes. When the pressure cooker has finished the cooking cycle, it will go the 'keep warm' cycle as the pressure drops. This will take about 5 minutes.

CHEFS NOTE

To serve, pour a ladle-full of sauce and spaghetti on each plate. Place a chicken breast on top and sprinkle with Parmesan cheese. Serve with a side of steamed broccoli for a delicious, healthy meal.

TURKEY TENDERLOIN WITH APPLES, SAGE AND STUFFING

498 calories per serving

Ingredients

- 1 tablespoon of extra-virgin olive oil
- 12-ounce turkey tenderloin - available in the fresh turkey meat section
- 2 cups stuffing
- 1½ cups of vegetable broth

- 2 slices turkey bacon – to place on top of the entire tenderloin
- 2 apples – cored and sliced
- 3 tablespoons chopped fresh sage

Method

1 In a preheated pressure cooker, add olive oil and turkey tenderloin. Brown it on all sides. Remove.

2 Pour in 2 cups of seasoned stuffing. Add the apples and the sage. Add the turkey tenderloin on top and place 2 slices of turkey bacon on top of the tenderloin. Pour vegetable broth over all. Lock the lid and set on high. Cook for 15 minutes on high pressure.

3 When the time is up, unplug the pressure cooker and let stand for 30 minutes.

4 Remove the lid and slice to serve. Pour broth over all.

CHEFS NOTE

Adding your own flavors using organic apples and fresh sage will fill your home with an amazing aroma. Plus turkey tenderloin cooks vey quickly.

TURKEY-SPINACH LASAGNA

485
calories per serving

Ingredients

- 2 tablespoons of extra-virgin olive oil
- 1 red onion, chopped
- 1 package of fresh spinach leaves
- 1 pound of ground turkey breast
- 1 pound of turkey sausage – removed from the casing
- Himalayan salt and fresh ground pepper to taste
- 1 jar of your favorite tomato sauce
- 1 12-ounce box of Pomi tomatoes

- (chopped)
- 1 tablespoon of tomato paste
- ¼ cup of water
- 1 cup feta
- 2 large eggs
- 2 garlic cloves, minced
- 1 teaspoon of Italian seasoning
- 1 package of no-boil lasagna noodles
- ¼ cup of Parmesan cheese – grated

Method

1 In an open pressure cooker, add the olive oil and heat at medium until it gets hot. Add the onion, ground turkey and sausage, Himalayan salt, and pepper and continue cooking until the onions become translucent and all the turkey meat is cooked. Add the tomato sauce, tomatoes, tomato paste and water to the turkey and onions. Stir and remove from heat and place in a large bowl.

2 In another bowl, mix feta, garlic, Italian seasoning and season with Himalayan salt and pepper.

3 Fill the bottom of your cooled pressure cooker with ¼ inch of water. Ladle some of the turkey meat and sauce into the bottom. Sprinkle with the feta mixture. Top with a layer of no-boil noodles. Repeat until all layers have been used. The final

layer should be the noodles that are topped with remaining sauce.

4 Lock the lid and bring to high pressure. Reduce heat to level to maintain high pressure and cook for 7 minutes.

5 After the 7 minutes, release the pressure and sprinkle with a little Parmesan. Cover and let the lasagna rest for at least 10 minutes before serving.

CHEFS NOTE

Look for ground, all-white meat turkey breast for the lowest fat version.

TURKEY MEATBALL STEW

474 calories per serving

Ingredients

- 1 pound of ground turkey
- 1 egg – lightly beaten
- ½ cup of Panko breadcrumbs
- 2 tablespoons of fresh parsley – minced
- 1 teaspoon of ground nutmeg
- 1 tablespoon of Worcestershire sauce
- 2 garlic cloves – minced
- Whole-grain flour for dusting

- 2 tablespoons of extra-virgin olive oil
- 1 cup of frozen peas
- ½ bag of small carrot sticks
- 6 fingerling potatoes
- ½ cup of chicken or vegetable stock
- ¼ cup of white wine
- 1 bay leaf

Method

1 In a large bowl, combine the turkey, egg, breadcrumbs, parsley, nutmeg, Worcestershire sauce, garlic and 1 tablespoon of the broth. Form into two-inch meatballs and dust them all lightly with the flour.

2 Heat the oil in the pressure cooker and add the meatballs. Cook them until they are brown on all sides.

3 Add the remaining ingredients. Lock the lid in place and bring the pressure to high. Cook for 5 minutes.

4 Allow the pressure to drop using the automatic release method and remove the lid. Discard the bay leaf and serve in bowls with some crusty, whole-grain bread.

CHEFS NOTE

This recipe can be prepared quickly using frozen turkey meatballs available in the freezer section of your local grocery store.

TURKEY CHILI WITH WHITE BEANS AND CORN BREAD

490 calories per serving

Ingredients

- 1 pound ground turkey breast or 3 cups of cooked chicken breast
- 1½ tablespoons of extra-virgin olive oil
- 1 red onion – chopped
- 4 garlic cloves – finely chopped
- 1 box of diced Pomi tomatoes or 6 Roma tomatoes – chopped
- 1 tablespoon of tomato paste
- 1 small can of diced green chilies
- 1 can of white or kidney beans – rinsed and drained
- 1 tablespoon of ground cumin
- 1 teaspoon of cayenne pepper
- 1 tablespoon of dried mustard
- 3 tablespoons of ketchup
- Himalayan sea salt and pepper to taste

Cornbread Topping:
- 1 cup of self-rising flour
- 1 cup of cornmeal
- ½ cup of almond milk
- 1 egg

Method

1 If you use ground turkey breast, cook it in a separate non-stick skillet while you cook the onions and garlic inside the pressure cooker in the olive oil for about 5 minutes.

2 Add all of the remaining ingredients, including the turkey or chicken.

3 Mix together the ingredients for the cornbread topping and pour over the turkey mixture. Lock the lid in place and cook for 45 minutes.

4 Turn the pressure cooker off and let the pressure drop down naturally. The pressure cooker will automatically go to the 'keep warm' setting.

CHEFS NOTE
Using a cornbread mix also works well. Simply follow label directions and cook the cornbread on top of the chili for a complete meal in your pressure cooker.

CHICKEN PICATTA

488 calories per serving

Ingredients

- 4 5-ounce boneless, skinless chicken breasts – pounded thin
- ½ cup of whole-grain flour
- ¼ cup extra-virgin olive oil
- 4 shallots – peeled and chopped
- 3 garlic cloves – minced
- 1 cup of chicken broth
-

- Juice of one lemon
- ½ cup of White Zinfandel or white wine
- Himalayan sea salt and pepper to taste
- 1 teaspoon of dried basil
- 7 ounces of angel hair pasta
- 1 head of broccoli – cut into pieces
- Slices of lemon for garnishing

Method

1 Pound chicken breasts and dust with flour. Heat the olive oil in the pressure cooker and cook chicken breasts (2 at a time) on each side for about 2 minutes. Remove and set aside.

2 Add the shallots and garlic and stir as you loosen the browned particles from the bottom of the pan. Stir in the broth, lemon juice, wine, sea salt, pepper and basil. Mix well.

3 Add the pasta, broccoli and cooked chicken breasts back to the pressure cooker.

4 Secure the lid. Bring the pressure up to medium-high heat and cook for 10 minutes. Release the pressure using the automatic pressure release and remove the lid.

5 Place chicken on a platter and cover to keep warm. To serve, pour sauce over chicken and angel hair and garnish with lemon slices.

6 Serve with fresh broccoli.

CHEFS NOTE
If you do not have potato starch, you can use flour to thicken the sauce.

CHICKEN BREAST PIQUANT WITH FINGERLING POTATOES

459 calories per serving

Ingredients

- ¾ cup of Rosé wine
- ½ low-sodium soy sauce
- ¼ cup of extra-virgin olive oil
- 2 tablespoons of water
- 1 clove of garlic
- 1 teaspoon of ground ginger

- ½ teaspoon of dried oregano
- 1 tablespoon of raw sugar or brown sugar
- 4 6-ounce boneless, skinless chicken breasts
- 8 fingerling potatoes
- 4 carrots – peeled and sliced

Method

1 In a blender, pour all ingredients in and blend well. Let stand for one hour.

2 Place chicken breasts, potatoes and carrots in your pressure cooker and pour the blended liquid over all.

3 Secure the lid in place and bring up to high pressure and let cook for 15 minutes.

4 Turn the pressure cooker off and let stand for about 10 minutes.

CHEFS NOTE

Fingerling potatoes cook quick and easy in a pressure cooker. Leave them whole or cut them in half.

ALMOND-CHICKEN MEATBALLS WITH LEMON SAUCE

SERVES 4

490 calories per serving

Ingredients

- ½ cup of whole-grain bread crumbs
- 1 cup almond milk
- 3 cups of raw ground chicken or turkey breast meat
- 1 tablespoon of extra-virgin olive oil
- 1 teaspoon of chopped parsley
- 1 egg - slightly beaten
- Himalayan sea salt and pepper to taste
- Pinch of nutmeg
- 1 egg - slightly beaten

- 1 cup of blanched slivered almonds – coarsely chopped
- 1½ cups of brown rice
- 4 carrots – peeled and sliced
- ½ cup of chicken broth
- 1 tablespoon of cornstarch
- 1 cup of Greek yogurt- plain
- ½ cup of chicken broth
- ½ teaspoon of fresh lemon peel – grated

Method

1 Soak the breadcrumbs in the almond milk for a few minutes and add the chicken or turkey meat. Mix well and add the olive oil, parsley, egg, sea salt, pepper and nutmeg. Chill thoroughly and form into 1-inch balls.

2 Roll the chicken balls in the slightly beaten egg, then in the crushed almonds. Place them in the pressure cooker with the brown rice, carrots and chicken broth. Secure the lid and bring the pressure up to high. Cook for 10 minutes. Let the pressure cooker go to the 'keep warm' stage.

3 While the chicken balls are cooking, mix the

cornstarch and Greek yogurt in a separate bowl. Stir into the chicken broth in a saucepan. Add the lemon peel and cook for five minutes.

4 Add the sauce to the chicken balls and serve warm.

CHEFS NOTE

For added flavor, toast the slivered almonds in a 375-degree oven for 10 minutes until they are golden brown. Then chop the toasted almonds or use a food processor to grind them.

44

Skinny
PRESSURE
COOKER MEAT

BEEF BOURGUIGNON

393
calories per serving

Ingredients

- 2 tablespoons of extra-virgin olive oil
- 2 red onions – diced
- 1 pound sliced Portabella mushrooms
- 2 cups of beef stew meat - cut into cubes
- 1 tablespoon of Red Wine Vinegar

- ¾ cup of Merlot or dry red wine
- 1 ¼ cup of beef broth
- Juice of half of a lemon
- Himalayan sea salt and pepper to taste for seasoning throughout

Method

1 Heat in the oil in the bottom of the pressure cooker and cook the onions and mushrooms for about five minutes. Season them with sea salt and pepper as they cook.

2 Move them to one side and add the beef to brown. Add vinegar, wine and beef broth and stir well. Lock the lid in place and bring to high pressure, then lower the heat and cook for 40 minutes.

3 When cooking is done, allow the pressure to drop using the automatic release method on your electric pressure cooker.

4 Serve over brown rice.

CHEFS NOTE

Another option is to cook the mushrooms and onions in a separate skillet until they are caramelized then add them to the beef mixture when cooking is done.

SWEET AND SOUR PORK CHOPS

490 calories per serving

Ingredients

- 4 2-inch thick pork chops
- ¼ cup of whole-grain flour
- 1½ tablespoons of extra-virgin olive oil
- ½ cup of organic Maple Syrup
- ½ cup of purified water
- ½ red onion - chopped

- 2 tablespoons of red wine vinegar
- 1 tablespoon of chili powder
- Pepper to taste
- 2 sweet potatoes – peeled and cut into squares
- 4 carrots – peeled and sliced

Method

1 Flour the pork chops and brown them in the olive oil in the bottom of your pressure cooker. In a separate bowl, combine the remaining ingredients and pour over the pork chops.

2 Secure the lid and set on high pressure. Cook for 15 minutes.

3 Let the pressure cooker go to the 'keep warm' phase and let the pressure come down naturally.

4 Remove the chops and place on a platter. Pour sauce over all. Enjoy!

CHEFS NOTE

Apple cider vinegar also works well in this recipe.

BEEF BRISKET IN BEER

360 calories per serving

Ingredients

- 1 4-pound brisket
- Himalayan sea salt and pepper to taste
- 1 red onion – sliced
- 1 cabbage - sliced
- ¼ cup of chili sauce
- 1 tablespoon of brown sugar
- 1 garlic clove – minced
- 12 ounces of beer
- 2 tablespoons of flour – optional
- ½ cup of water – optional

Method

1 Trim the excess fat from the brisket and season with the sea salt and pepper. Place the meat in the bottom of the pressure cooker. Cover with the onion slices and cabbage.

2 In a separate bowl, combine the chili sauce, sugar, garlic and beer. Pour over the brisket.

3 Secure the lid and bring it up to high pressure. Let it cook for 40 minutes. Let the pressure go to the 'keep warm' phase. Remove the lid.

CHEFS NOTE

If you would like to make gravy, pour off the liquid into a saucepan. Mix the flour and water together and pour into the pan drippings. Stir until thick and bubbly.

ONE-POT SPAGHETTI

495
calories per
serving

Ingredients

- 1 pound of ground beef
- 10 ounces of pasta (made from vegetables – broken into pieces)
- 1 small onion – chopped
- 2 tablespoons of extra-virgin olive oil
- 1 small red or green pepper – chopped
- 1 box of Pomi tomatoes
- Himalayan sea salt and pepper to taste

Method

1 Combine all the ingredients in the pressure cooker.

2 Secure the lid and heat to high pressure. Cook for 15 minutes.

3 Lower the heat and let simmer for about 10 minutes.

4 Remove the lid and serve.

CHEFS NOTE

Look for pasta made from vegetables, available in the pasta section of your local grocery store. It is gluten-free, tastes delicious and will not make you feel bloated.

POT ROAST

498 calories per serving

Ingredients

- 1 tablespoon of extra-virgin olive oil
- 1 4-pound roast beef
- Himalayan sea salt and pepper to taste
- 1 teaspoon of celery seed
- 1 teaspoon of dried oregano

- ½ cup of water
- 2 tablespoons of apple cider vinegar
- 1 medium onion – chopped
- 8 fingerling potatoes
- 4 carrots – peeled and sliced

Method

1 In the bottom of the pressure cooker, heat the oil and brown the roast on all sides. Add all the seasonings.

2 Combine the water and the vinegar and pour over the roast. Place the onions on top and add the potatoes and carrots.

3 Secure the lid and bring the pressure up to high. Cook for 40 minutes.

4 Once the cooking is done, let it come down to the 'keep warm' phase and let sit for about 20 minutes.

5 Slice and serve.

CHEFS NOTE

You can make delicious gravy with the juices from the meat that collect at the bottom of the pressure cooker. Remove the meat and let stand covered with foil. Mix together ¼ cup of water with 1 tablespoon of potato starch or whole-grain flour. Add to the liquid in the pressure cooker and stir well as you heat through to bubbly gravy. Serve the pot roast with the gravy.

CUBAN BEEF WITH RED CABBAGE

430
calories per serving

Ingredients

- 1 large garlic clove – finely chopped
- 1 4-pound sirloin beef tip roast
- 1 red cabbage - sliced
- 1 package of dry spaghetti sauce mix
- 1 box of Pomi chopped tomatoes
- 1 cup of red wine – Merlot or Cabernet Sauvignon works well

- 1½ tablespoons of extra-virgin olive oil
- 3 medium size zucchini - chopped
- 1 large red pepper - chopped
- 1 small container of sliced Portabella mushrooms – sliced
- 1 teaspoon of garlic powder
- Himalayan sea salt and pepper to taste

Method

1 Place garlic on the bottom of the pressure cooker. Place the meat and cabbage on the garlic and sprinkle with the spaghetti sauce mix. Add the chopped tomatoes and red wine.

2 Secure the lid and bring up to high pressure and cook for 30 minutes. Release the pressure with the automatic pressure release and keep warm while you cook the vegetables.

3 Fifteen minutes before the roast is done, sauté the zucchini, red pepper and mushrooms in olive oil. Season with garlic powder, sea salt and pepper – serve with the roast.

CHEFS NOTE
Create delicious gravy using the juice from the meat in the bottom of the pressure cooker. Simply thicken with 1 teaspoon of tomato paste.

HAWAIIAN SHISH KEBABS

486
calories per
serving

Ingredients

- 1½ pounds of top sirloin – cut into 1-inch squares
- 1½ cups of brown rice
- ½ cup of low-sodium soy sauce
- 1 tablespoon of sugar-in-the-raw
- 2 tablespoons of extra-virgin olive oil
- 1 teaspoon of ground ginger
- Pepper to taste

- 2 garlic cloves – minced
- 1 small container of fresh whole Portabella mushrooms
- 1 small container of whole fresh cherry tomatoes
- 4 small red onions – quartered
- 2 large red peppers – cut into large square pieces

Method

1 Combine the soy sauce, sugar-in-the-raw, olive oil, ginger, pepper and garlic – mix well and set aside.

2 Pour rice in the bottom of the pressure cooker. Place a cherry tomato on a skewer, followed by onion, meat, red pepper and mushroom. REPEAT until skewer is full. Place each skewer in the pressure cooker. Pour the soy sauce mixture over all.

3 Secure the lid and bring up to high pressure. Cook for 15 minutes.

4 Once cooking is complete, use the automatic pressure release to open lid. Serve immediately or keep warm for serving at a party.

CHEFS NOTE

Other vegetables can be used on the skewer such as zucchini, yellow squash or yellow peppers.

BAKED PEPPER STEAK

490 calories per serving

Ingredients

- 4 6-ounce sirloin steaks – about 2-inches thick
- Prepared mustard
- 8 fingerling potatoes
- 1 red onion – sliced
- 1 small container of Portabella mushrooms – sliced
- 1 red pepper – sliced
- 2 tablespoons of Worcestershire sauce
- 1 cup of chili sauce
- Himalayan sea salt and pepper to taste
- Paprika to taste

Method

1 Spread mustard on both sides of each steak. Place in the bottom of the pressure cooker.

2 Cover the steaks with potatoes, onions, mushrooms and red pepper. Add the Worcestershire sauce, chili sauce, salt, pepper and paprika.

3 Secure the lid and bring up to high pressure. Cook for 20 minutes and turn to automatic pressure release.

4 Let the steaks rest for about 10 minutes. Pour remaining sauce over each steak and serve.

CHEFS NOTE

Keep these ingredients on hand so you can always make a quick dinner any night of the week in your electric pressure cooker.

GROUND BEEF AND WINE

484
calories per serving

Ingredients

- 1½ tablespoons of extra-virgin olive oil
- ½ red onion – sliced
- 1 garlic clove – minced
- 1 small container of sliced Portabella mushrooms
- 1 pound of ground chuck beef
- ½ cup of Burgundy wine
- Juice of one lemon
- 1½ cups of beef consommé – from a box
- Himalayan sea salt and pepper to taste
- 2 cups of brown rice or 1 cup of pasta
- 1 cup of plain Greek yogurt
- Parsley for garnish

Method

1 Heat oil in the bottom of the pressure cooker and cook the onion, garlic and mushrooms. Add the ground chuck and cook until no longer pink.

2 Add the red wine, lemon juice, consommé, sea salt and pepper to taste, brown rice and yogurt.

3 Secure the lid and bring up to high pressure. Cook for 10 minutes.

4 Turn to automatic pressure release and let it go to 'keep warm.' It is ready to serve with some crusty French bread.

CHEFS NOTE

Plain Greek yogurt works well in place of sour cream that saves both calories and fat. Plus it is delicious.

SHERRY PORK CHOPS WITH APPLES

499
calories per serving

Ingredients

- 1½ tablespoons of extra-virgin olive oil
- 4 6-ounce pork chops
- 1½ cups of brown rice
- 3 medium apples – sliced
- ¼ cup brown sugar
- 1 teaspoon of cinnamon
- 2 tablespoons of butter
- Himalayan sea salt and pepper to taste
- 1 cup Sherry wine

Method

1 Heat oil in the bottom of the pressure cooker and brown pork chops on both sides. Remove them from the pressure cooker.

2 Pour the brown rice in the bottom of the pressure cooker and place the sliced apples on top. Sprinkle with the brown sugar and cinnamon. Dot with butter and place the pork chops on top of the apples. Pour the Sherry wine over all.

3 Secure the lid and bring up to high pressure. Cook for 20 minutes. Release the pressure with the automatic pressure release and keep warm for about 10 minutes. Serve.

CHEFS NOTE

Honey Crisp or Pink Lady apples work well with this recipe.

SERVES 4

STEAK DIANE WITH PORTABELLA MUSHROOMS

498 calories per serving

Ingredients

- 4 6-ounce steak filets – pounded thin
- Himalayan sea salt and pepper to taste
- 2 tablespoons of extra-virgin olive oil
- 2 tablespoons of low-sodium soy sauce
- 1½ cups of beef broth – from a box
- 2 tablespoons of Dijon mustard
- 1 tablespoon of cornstarch
- 3 shallots – diced
- 1 small container of sliced Portabella mushrooms
- 8 fingerling potatoes

Method

1 Season each filet with sea salt and pepper. Coat with olive oil and soy sauce – roll up and set aside.

2 In a separate bowl, combine the broth, mustard and cornstarch – mix well. Heat pressure cooker, unroll each steak and brown them on each side for about 1 minute – remove and set aside.

3 Cook the shallots and mushrooms for about 2 minutes. Add the potatoes and steak back to the pressure cooker and pour the broth mixture over all.

4 Secure the lid and bring up to high pressure. Cook for 10 minutes. After cooking is complete, turn to automatic pressure release. Remove lid and serve.

CHEFS NOTE

If fingerling potatoes are not available, substitute small new red potatoes. You can also carrots or broccoli to the pressure cooker for a complete meal.

Skinny
PRESSURE
COOKER VEGETABLES

ARTICHOKES IN BEER WITH TOFU

SERVES 4

352 calories per serving

Ingredients

- 4 fresh artichokes
- 1 12-ounce bottle of light beer
- 1 small container of Portabella mushrooms – sliced
- 8 ounces of tofu – cut into chunks

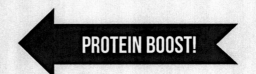

PROTEIN BOOST!

Method

1 Wash and remove the bottom leaves from the artichokes and cut off any thorns. Remove the fuzzy choke from the center and stuff the center firmly with the mushrooms. Place them right side up in the bottom of your pressure cooker. Pour the beer over all of the artichokes and add the tofu.

2 Secure the lid and bring the pressure up to high. Cook for 10 minutes. Turn back to automatic pressure release and remove the lid to serve.

CHEFS NOTE

To save calories, use light beer, however regular beer can be used. The tofu absorbs the flavor of the beer for an added protein source.

VEGETABLE-SWEET POTATO CASSEROLE

349 calories per serving

Ingredients

- 1 bunch of fresh asparagus
- 2 sweet potatoes – peeled and sliced
- 1 red onion – sliced
- 1½ cups of sliced Portabella mushrooms
- For Sauce:
- 2 tablespoons of extra-virgin olive oil
- ¼ cup whole-grain flour
- 1½ cups of chicken broth – from a box or homemade
- 1 cup of plain Greek yogurt
- Juice of one lemon

Method

1 Place the vegetables in layers in the bottom of the electric pressure cooker. Combine the ingredients for the sauce and pour over all.

2 Secure the lid and bring up to high pressure. Cook for 10 minutes for tender vegetables and 5 minutes for al dente. Serve.

CHEFS NOTE

This recipe works well with many vegetables. Try broccoli, cauliflower or whatever is in season.

SAVORY SPINACH DIP

SERVES 4

173 calories per serving

Ingredients

- 1 cup of plain Greek yogurt
- 1 package of dry Parmesan salad dressing mix
- 2 packages of frozen chopped spinach – defrosted and well-drained or 2 bags of fresh organic spinach – chopped

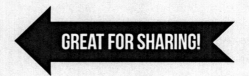

GREAT FOR SHARING!

Method

1 Place the spinach in the pressure cooker. Combine the Greek yogurt with the salad dressing mix and pour over spinach – mix well.

2 Secure lid and bring up to high pressure. Cook for 5 minutes. Use the automatic pressure release to bring the pressure down and serve immediately.

CHEFS NOTE
Add chopped artichokes or onion for an added twist to this simple recipe.

COOKED RED CABBAGE

38 calories per ½ cup serving

Ingredients

- 1 head of red cabbage – sliced
- 2 tablespoons of extra-virgin olive oil
- Juice of 1 lemon
- ½ cup of red wine vinegar
- 1 teaspoon of sugar-in-the-raw

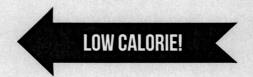
LOW CALORIE!

Method

1 Cut the cabbage slices into small pieces and place inside the pressure cooker. Cover with the remaining ingredients.

2 Secure the lid and bring up to high pressure. Cook for 10 minutes. Use the automatic pressure release to release the pressure and remove the lid. Serve immediately.

CHEFS NOTE

This stores well in the refrigerator to reheat again for future meals.

GREEN BEAN CASSEROLE

168
calories per ½
cup serving

Ingredients

- 2 tablespoons of extra-virgin olive oil
- 1 small container of button mushrooms – chopped
- ½ yellow onion – chopped
- ¼ cup whole-grain flour
- 1 cup of plain almond milk
- 1 cup of plain Greek yogurt
- 6 ounces of 2% sharp cheese – grated
- A few drops of Tabasco sauce

- 1 teaspoon of soy sauce
- Pepper to taste
- Pinch of Lawry's seasoned salt
- 3 8-ounce packages of frozen French-cut green beans
- 1 8-ounce can of water chestnuts, drained and sliced
- ½ cup of slivered almonds – toast in the oven at 375 degrees for 8 minutes.

Method

1 Heat the oil in the pressure cooker and cook the mushrooms and onions for about 3 minutes. Remove.

2 Stir in flour until smooth. Add the almond milk and yogurt; cook until thick. Add the cheese, Tabasco, soy sauce, seasoned salt, pepper and beans. Mix well and add the chestnuts.

3 Secure the lid and bring up to high pressure. Cook for 8 minutes. Use the automatic pressure release to release the pressure and keep warm.

4 Sprinkle with the toasted almonds.

CHEFS NOTE

While the beans are cooking in the pressure cooker, toast the almonds. You can toast an entire bag of slivered almonds and store in an airtight container to sprinkle over other vegetables and salads for extra flavor and crunch.

MINT-GLAZED BABY CARROTS

110 calories per ½ cup serving

Ingredients

- 2 tablespoons of extra-virgin olive oil
- 1 tablespoon of light brown sugar
- 2 tablespoons of raw honey
- 1/8 of a teaspoon of peppermint extract
- 3 cups of baby carrots
- 1 tablespoon of fresh mint leaves – chopped or 1½ teaspoon of dried mint leaves

Method

1 Heat the oil in the bottom of the pressure cooker and add the brown sugar, honey and peppermint extract. Stir well and add the carrots, coating them thoroughly.

2 Secure the lid and bring up to high pressure. Cook for 5 minutes.

3 Release the pressure using the automatic pressure release and open the lid. Remove the carrots to a serving bowl and sprinkle with fresh mint.

CHEFS NOTE

This recipe also works well with sliced carrots, if you prefer them to whole ones. The cooking time can be reduced by one minute.

DUTCH EGGPLANT

237 calories per serving

Ingredients

- 1 2-pound eggplant – peeled and diced
- ½ yellow onion – chopped
- ½ of a red pepper – chopped
- 2 tablespoons of extra-virgin olive oil
- 1 10-ounce box of tomato soup
- Pepper to taste

Method

1 Cook eggplant, onions and red pepper in olive oil for 2 minutes in the bottom of the pressure cooker. Add the soup and pepper to taste. Seal the lid and turn up to high pressure. Cook for 5 minutes.

2 Reduce the pressure with the automatic pressure release and remove the lid. Serve immediately.

CHEFS NOTE

Soup in a cardboard box is readily available in most health food sections of local grocery stores. Experiment with other soup flavors such as butternut squash or vegetable broth.

SWEET POTATOES WITH APRICOTS

160 calories per ½ cup serving

Ingredients

- 4 medium-size sweet potatoes – peeled and cut in half
- A pinch of Himalayan sea salt
- 1 teaspoon of cinnamon
- 1 teaspoon of orange peel – shredded
- 4 apricots – peeled and cut into quarters
- 2 tablespoons of extra-virgin olive oil
- ½ cup pecan halves

Method

1 Place sweet potatoes in the bottom of the pressure cooker. Sprinkle with sea salt, cinnamon and orange peel. Place apricots over the top and drizzle olive oil over all. Sprinkle with pecan halves.

2 Secure the lid and bring up to high pressure. Cook for 10 minutes.

3 Release the pressure using the automatic pressure release and keep warm until ready to serve.

CHEFS NOTE

Another option is to toast the pecans in a 375-degree oven and sprinkle them over the cooked sweet potatoes for more of a crunch and a toasted flavor.

HERBED TOMATOES

70
calories per
serving

Ingredients

- 4 ripe tomatoes
- Himalayan sea salt and pepper to taste
- 1 teaspoon dried thyme or marjoram

- ¼ cup parsley – chopped
- ¼ cup extra-virgin olive oil
- ¼ Tarragon vinegar

Method

1 Cut the top of each tomato and place them in the bottom of the pressure cooker – sprinkle sea salt, pepper, thyme and parsley on the top of each tomato.

2 Combine the olive oil and vinegar and drizzle over the top.

3 Secure the lid and bring up to high pressure. Cook for 5 minutes. Release the pressure using the automatic pressure release. Serve immediately.

CHEFS NOTE
Add more flavors to the tomatoes using fresh thyme or marjoram.

MASHED POTATO CAULIFLOWER

80 calories per serving

Ingredients

- 1 head of cauliflower – preferably organic
- 1 teaspoon of garlic powder
- Himalayan sea salt and pepper to taste
- 1 tablespoon of extra-virgin olive oil

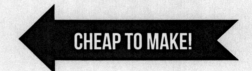

CHEAP TO MAKE!

Method

1 Cut off the base of the cauliflower and place inside the pressure cooker. Season with garlic powder, sea salt and pepper – secure the lid and bring up to high pressure. Cook for 5 minutes.

2 Release the pressure with the automatic pressure release and remove the lid.

3 Place the cauliflower in a food processor and process until the desired consistency is achieved.

4 Serve immediately.

CHEFS NOTE
The longer you blend, the smoother the cauliflower will become for a creamy mashed potato texture.

Skinny
PRESSURE
COOKER DESSERTS

DARK CHOCOLATE PUDDING IN A JAR

410 calories per serving

Ingredients

- ½ cup of Sugar-In-The-Raw
- ½ cup of Butter and Olive Oil (available in the butter section of the grocery store)
- 2 eggs - beaten
- ½ cup of flour
- ½ teaspoon of sea salt
- 1 teaspoon of baking powder
- 1 teaspoon of vanilla extract
- 4 squares of dark chocolate – melted
- 4 teaspoons of seedless, raspberry jam
- Fresh raspberries

Method

1 In an electric mixing bowl, cream the sugar with the butter/olive oil and add the eggs, flour, sea salt, baking powder, vanilla and melted dark chocolate.

2 Butter 5 mini-jars or ramekins and put a tablespoon of raspberry jam in each jar. Divide the batter between 4 mini jars or ramekins, put the lids on or cover them with plastic wrap and freeze.

3 When you are ready to use them, remove the lids and cover loosely with greased tin foil. Place them in your pressure cooker with 4½ cups of water and set the STEAM timer for 35 minutes.

4 When the timer goes off, release immediately, remove them from the steamer and let cool a few minutes. Top with fresh raspberries and serve immediately.

CHEFS NOTE

Look for good dark chocolate in the candy aisle or gourmet food section of your local grocery store.

RHUBARB CRUNCH

370
calories per
serving

Ingredients

- 1 cup sifted whole-grain flour
- 1 cup of oatmeal
- ½ cup of brown sugar
- ½ cup of chopped nuts
- 2 tablespoons of butter and olive oil (available in the butter section)

- 3 cups of diced rhubarb – fresh or frozen
- ¼ cup of Sugar-In-The-Raw
- 1 teaspoon of cinnamon

Method

1 Combine flour, oatmeal, brown sugar and nuts. Cut in the butter with a pastry cutter until a crumbly mixture forms. Spread half of the oatmeal mixture in the bottom of the electric pressure cooker.

2 Mix the rhubarb with the raw sugar and cinnamon. Pour directly over the dry ingredients. Top with the remaining half of dry mixture.

3 Secure the lid and bring up to high pressure. Cook for 15 minutes.

4 Release the pressure using the automatic pressure release. Remove the lid and serve.

CHEFS NOTE
Other fruits work well with this recipe – such as strawberries, blueberries, apricots and cherries.

FRUIT COMPOTE

290
calories per
serving

Ingredients

- 3 half-pints of raspberries
- 2 half-pints of blueberries
- ¼ cup of sugar-in-the-raw

- 2 tablespoons of Chambord (raspberry liqueur – optional)
- 2 pints of vanilla ice cream

Method

1 Combine the raspberries, blueberries, raw sugar, and Chambord in the pressure cooker. Bring it up to a high pressure and cook for 5 minutes.

2 Release the pressure with the automatic pressure release and ladle the fruit over a scoop of ice cream.

CHEFS NOTE
Choose organic fruit whenever possible to avoid the pesticides which are so commonplace.

DARK CHOCOLATE BREAD PUDDING

377 calories per serving

Ingredients

- 1 loaf of Italian bread – cut into chunks
- 2 cups of vanilla almond milk
- ¼ cup vanilla Greek yogurt
- 2 tablespoons of instant coffee or ½ cup of coffee liqueur
- 1 cup sugar-in-the-raw
- 1 cup of brown sugar
- ¼ cup dark cocoa powder
- 1 tablespoon of vanilla extract
- 2 teaspoons of pure almond extract
- 2 teaspoons of ground cinnamon
- 6 large eggs – beaten
- 1 cup of dark chocolate chips

Method

1 Place bread inside the pressure cooker. In a large bowl, whisk together the almond milk, Greek yogurt and coffee.

2 In another bowl, combine both sugars and cocoa powder. Mix well. Add this mixture to the milk mixture and whisk together until thoroughly blended.

3 Add both extracts and cinnamon to the beaten eggs. Combine the egg mixture with the milk mixture. Stir in the chocolate chips. Pour the mixture over the bread cubes.

4 Let the bread soak for about 20 minutes.

5 Secure the lid and bring the pressure up to high. Cook for 20 minutes. Allow the pressure to drop using the automatic pressure release.

6 Remove the lid and let it cool for a few minutes. Serve warm.

CHEFS NOTE
Individual ramekins may be used and cooked right inside the pressure cooker. Fresh raspberries or sliced strawberries work well for a garnish.

CARAMEL FLAN

300 calories per serving

Ingredients

- ¾ cup of sugar-in-the-raw
- ¼ cup of water
- 3 whole eggs and 2 egg yolks
- Pinch of Himalayan sea salt
- 2 cups of vanilla almond milk
- 1 teaspoon of vanilla extract
- 4 tablespoons of caramel syrup

Method

1 In a bowl, whisk together sugar, water, eggs and egg yolks. Add a pinch of salt, milk and vanilla extract. Mix well.

2 Pour a tablespoon of caramel syrup into individual ramekins. Pour the egg mixture into each ramekin so they are ¾ full. Cover with foil.

3 Pour 1½ cups of water into the pressure cooker. Place the stand inside and set the ramekins on top. Secure lid and bring up to high pressure. Cook for 6 minutes.

4 Use a natural pressure release for 10 minutes and then do a quick release with the automatic pressure release function.

5 Remove the ramekins carefully and let them cool uncovered.

6 When cool, refrigerate for at least 4 hours before serving.

7 Serve with chopped hazelnuts.

CHEFS NOTE
Substitute hazelnut syrup for caramel syrup for a change in this recipe.

CHOCOLATE-CHIP CHEESECAKE

490 calories per serving

Ingredients

Ingredients for the crust:
- ¾ package of Oreo cookies – ground in a food processor or blender

Ingredients For The Filling:
- ½ cup sugar
- 2 eggs
- 3 packages of cream cheese
- ½ cup of mini-chips
- ¼ cup chocolate syrup
- 1 tablespoon of lemon juice
- 1 teaspoon of grated lemon zest
- 1 teaspoon of vanilla extract
- ¼ cup of mini-chips

Method

1 Press the cookie crumbs in the bottom of a spring-form pan. Place a long sheet of aluminium foil one direction and place another piece of foil on top to form a cross. Place the spring-form pan in the middle. Fold the edges down a bit so they can be used as handles to bring out of the pressure cooker.

2 Using an electric mixer, beat eggs and sugar for 5 minutes. Add cream cheese, one package at a time and blend well.

3 Add the remaining ingredients and pour into the spring-form pan. Sprinkle with mini-chips.

4 Place the foil-lined pan inside the pressure cooker. Secure the lid and bring up to high pressure. Cook for 15 minutes.

5 Turn off the heat and allow the pressure to come down naturally. Remove the lid and let the steam subside before removing the cheesecake from the pressure cooker.

6 Set on a wire rack to cool for at least one hour.

7 Place in refrigerator and chill for at least 6-8 hours. Release the cheesecake from the spring-form pan and serve.

CHEFS NOTE
Garnish with fresh raspberries for a dazzling dessert.

EASY RICE PUDDING WITH RAISINS

SERVES 4

440 calories per serving

Ingredients

- 1 cup of white rice (uncooked)
- ½ cup of sugar-in-the-raw
- 5 cups of vanilla almond milk
- 1 teaspoon of vanilla extract
- 1 teaspoon of ground cinnamon
- ¾ cup of raisins

Method

1 Add all the ingredients to the pressure cooker and mix well. Secure the lid and bring up to high pressure. Then turn it down to low heat and cook for 25 minutes.

2 Release the pressure using the automatic pressure release. Enjoy hot or cold.

CHEFS NOTE

In place of cinnamon, you could add ground nutmeg or cardamom. Almond extract may be used in place of vanilla extract for a change.

PUMPKIN BREAD PUDDING

445 calories per serving

Ingredients

- 2/3 cup of solid packed pumpkin
- 6 slices of cinnamon-raisin bread – cut into chunks
- Cooking spray
- ½ cup of Sugar-In-The-Raw
- 3 large eggs

- 1 cup of vanilla almond milk
- 1 teaspoon of vanilla extract
- A pinch of Himalayan sea salt
- 1/8 of a teaspoon of ground nutmeg
- 2 cups of water

Method

1 Use a baking dish that can fit inside your pressure cooker and spray the inside of the baking dish with cooking spray. Place the bread chunks inside the baking dish.

2 Whisk together the sugar and eggs. Add the milk, vanilla extract, salt and nutmeg. Mix well and pour over the bread. Make sure all the bread is covered with the liquid. Cover tightly with aluminium foil so no water can get inside.

3 Pour 2 cups of water into the pressure cooker. Place the baking dish on a stand inside the pressure cooker. Secure the lid and bring up to high pressure. Reduce it to low heat and cook for 20 minutes.

4 Release the pressure using the automatic pressure release. Pour off any water that might have accumulated on the top of the aluminium foil and remove it.

5 Let the bread pudding rest for about 10 minutes and serve warm.

CHEFS NOTE

Bread pudding holds up well in the refrigerator for several days. Warm it up in the oven to serve.

STUFFED APPLES

231
calories per serving

Ingredients

- 4 apples
- ¼ cup of raisins
- ¼ cup of chopped nuts

- ½ teaspoon of grated orange rind
- 1 teaspoon of cinnamon
- 1 tablespoon of melted butter

Method

1 Core each apple and set aside. Combine the remaining ingredients and spoon the filling into each apple. Place the apples inside the pressure cooker. Secure the lid and bring up to high pressure. Cook for 10 minutes.

2 Release the pressure with the automatic pressure release and let stand for 5 minutes. Remove the lid and serve immediately.

CHEFS NOTE
Lemon rind also works well in place of orange rind. You could also add a pinch of nutmeg to the mixture for added flavor.

CHOCOLATE PEANUT BUTTER CAKE

435 calories per serving

Ingredients

- 1 cup of whole-grain flour
- 1/3 cup of sugar-in-the-raw
- 2 tablespoons of cocoa powder
- 1 ½ teaspoon of baking powder
- ½ cup of chocolate-almond milk
- 2 tablespoons of extra-virgin olive oil
- 2 teaspoons of vanilla extract

- ½ cup of peanut butter chips
- ½ cup of chocolate-chips
- ½ cup of peanuts – roughly chopped
- ¾ cup of Sugar-In-The-Raw
- 2 tablespoons of cocoa powder
- 1½ cups of boiling water

Method

1 Lightly coat the inside of the pressure cooker with cooking spray and set aside.

2 In a separate bowl, stir together the flour, sugar, cocoa powder and baking powder. Add the milk, olive oil and vanilla extract. Stir to moisten. Gently fold in both chips and peanuts. Spread the batter evenly inside the pressure cooker.

3 In another bowl, mix together ¾ cup of the raw sugar, cocoa powder and boiling water. Pour over the ingredients in the pressure cooker. Secure the lid and bring up to high pressure. Cook for 40 minutes.

4 Release the pressure with the automatic pressure release. Remove the lid and let stand for 10 minutes.

5 Do not leave the cake on the 'keep warm' as this will dry it out.

6 Spoon into dessert bowls and serve by itself or with a scoop of ice cream. Enjoy!

CHEFS NOTE

Look for real peanut butter chips instead of artificially flavored peanut butter pieces.

PRESSURE COOKER APPLE PIE

420 calories per serving

Ingredients

- Cooking spray
- 8 apples – peeled and sliced
- 2 teaspoons of ground cinnamon
- ½ teaspoon of allspice
- ½ teaspoon of nutmeg
- ¾ cup of almond milk
- 2 tablespoons of butter – softened
- ¾ cup of sugar-in-the-raw

- 2 eggs
- 1 teaspoon of vanilla extract
- ½ cup of Bisquick mix

Topping Ingredients:
- 1 cup of Bisquick
- 1/3 cup of brown sugar
- 3 tablespoons of butter

Method

1 Lightly coat the inside of the pressure cooker with cooking spray. Toss the apples with all the spices and place inside the pressure cooker.

2 In a bowl combine the milk, butter, sugar, eggs, vanilla extract and Bisquick. Pour this mixture over the apples.

3 In a separate bowl, combine 1 cup of the Bisquick and brown sugar. Cut butter into the mixture until it crumbles. Sprinkle this mixture on top of the pie mixture inside the pressure cooker.

4 Secure the lid and bring up to high pressure. Cook for 20 minutes.

5 Release the pressure with the automatic pressure release. Open the lid and serve immediately.

CHEFS NOTE

Raw honey can replace the sugar-in-the-raw with the juice of half of a lemon. For a quick shortcut, use ready-made apple pie filling for the apple mixture that is first placed in the pressure cooker however this may increase the overall calorie count of the dish.

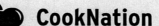 CookNation

Other
COOKNATION
TITLES

If you enjoyed 'The Skinny Pressure Cooker Cookbook' we'd really appreciate your feedback. Reviews help others decide if this is the right book for them.

Thank you.

You may also be interested in other '**Skinny**' titles in the CookNation series. You can find all the following great titles by searching under '**CookNation**'.

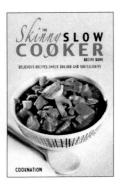

THE SKINNY SLOW COOKER RECIPE BOOK

Delicious Recipes Under 300, 400 And 500 Calories.

Paperback / eBook

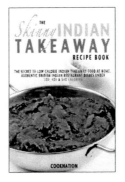

THE SKINNY INDIAN TAKEAWAY RECIPE BOOK

Authentic British Indian Restaurant Dishes Under 300, 400 And 500 Calories. The Secret To Low Calorie Indian Takeaway Food At Home.

Paperback / eBook

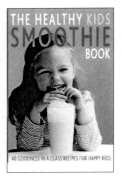

THE HEALTHY KIDS SMOOTHIE BOOK

40 Delicious Goodness In A Glass Recipes for Happy Kids.

eBook

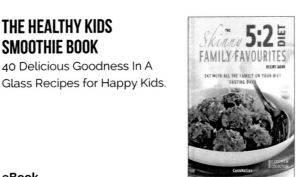

THE SKINNY 5:2 FAST DIET FAMILY FAVOURITES RECIPE BOOK

Eat With All The Family On Your Diet Fasting Days.

Paperback / eBook

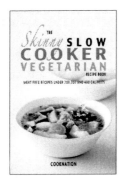

THE SKINNY SLOW COOKER VEGETARIAN RECIPE BOOK

40 Delicious Recipes Under 200, 300 And 400 Calories.

Paperback / eBook

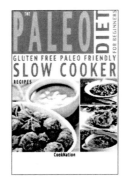

THE PALEO DIET FOR BEGINNERS SLOW COOKER RECIPE BOOK

Gluten Free, Everyday Essential Slow Cooker Paleo Recipes For Beginners.

eBook

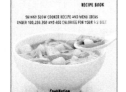

THE SKINNY 5:2 SLOW COOKER RECIPE BOOK

Skinny Slow Cooker Recipe And Menu Ideas Under 100, 200, 300 & 400 Calories For Your 5:2 Diet.

Paperback / eBook

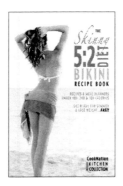

THE SKINNY 5:2 BIKINI DIET RECIPE BOOK

Recipes & Meal Planners Under 100, 200 & 300 Calories. Get Ready For Summer & Lose Weight...FAST!

Paperback / eBook

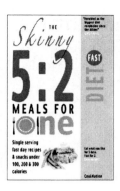

THE SKINNY 5:2 FAST DIET MEALS FOR ONE

Single Serving Fast Day Recipes & Snacks Under 100, 200 & 300 Calories.

Paperback / eBook

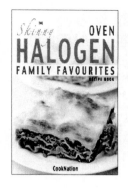

THE SKINNY HALOGEN OVEN FAMILY FAVOURITES RECIPE BOOK

Healthy, Low Calorie Family Meal-Time Halogen Oven Recipes Under 300, 400 and 500 Calories.

Paperback / eBook

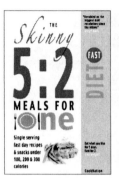

THE SKINNY 5:2 FAST DIET VEGETARIAN MEALS FOR ONE

Single Serving Fast Day Recipes & Snacks Under 100, 200 & 300 Calories.

Paperback / eBook

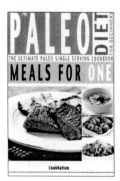

THE PALEO DIET FOR BEGINNERS MEALS FOR ONE

The Ultimate Paleo Single Serving Cookbook.

Paperback / eBook

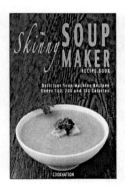

THE SKINNY SOUP MAKER RECIPE BOOK

Delicious Low Calorie, Healthy and Simple Soup Recipes Under 100, 200 and 300 Calories. Perfect For Any Diet and Weight Loss Plan.

Paperback / eBook

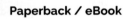

THE PALEO DIET FOR BEGINNERS HOLIDAYS

Thanksgiving, Christmas & New Year Paleo Friendly Recipes.
eBook

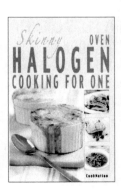

SKINNY HALOGEN OVEN COOKING FOR ONE

Single Serving, Healthy, Low Calorie Halogen Oven RecipesUnder 200, 300 and 400 Calories.

Paperback / eBook

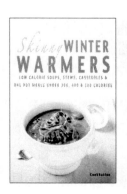

SKINNY WINTER WARMERS RECIPE BOOK

Soups, Stews, Casseroles & One Pot Meals Under 300, 400 & 500 Calories.

Paperback / eBook

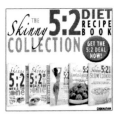

THE SKINNY 5:2 DIET RECIPE BOOK COLLECTION

All The 5:2 Fast Diet Recipes You'll Ever Need. All Under 100, 200, 300, 400 And 500 Calories.

eBook

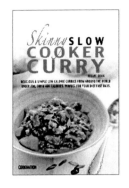

THE SKINNY SLOW COOKER CURRY RECIPE BOOK

Low Calorie Curries From Around The World.

Paperback / eBook

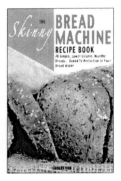

THE SKINNY BREAD MACHINE RECIPE BOOK

70 Simple, Lower Calorie, Healthy Breads...Baked To Perfection In Your Bread Maker.

Paperback / eBook

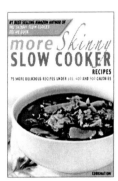

MORE SKINNY SLOW COOKER RECIPES

75 More Delicious Recipes Under 300, 400 & 500 Calories.

Paperback / eBook

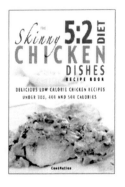

THE SKINNY 5:2 DIET CHICKEN DISHES RECIPE BOOK

Delicious Low Calorie Chicken Dishes Under 300, 400 & 500 Calories.

Paperback / eBook

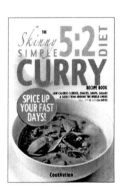

THE SKINNY 5:2 CURRY RECIPE BOOK

Spice Up Your Fast Days With Simple Low Calorie Curries, Snacks, Soups, Salads & Sides Under 200, 300 & 400 Calories.

Paperback / eBook

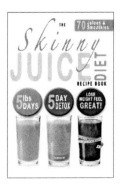

THE SKINNY JUICE DIET RECIPE BOOK

5lbs, 5 Days. The Ultimate Kick- Start Diet and Detox Plan to Lose Weight & Feel Great!

Paperback / eBook

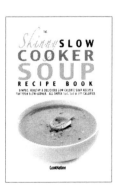

THE SKINNY SLOW COOKER SOUP RECIPE BOOK

Simple, Healthy & Delicious Low Calorie Soup Recipes For Your Slow Cooker. All Under 100, 200 & 300 Calories.

Paperback / eBook

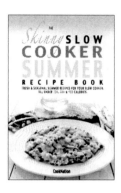

THE SKINNY SLOW COOKER SUMMER RECIPE BOOK

Fresh & Seasonal Summer Recipes For Your Slow Cooker. All Under 300, 400 And 500 Calories.

Paperback / eBook

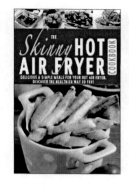

THE SKINNY HOT AIR FRYER COOKBOOK

Delicious & Simple Meals For Your Hot Air Fryer: Discover The Healthier Way To Fry.

Paperback / eBook

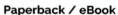

THE SKINNY ACTIFRY COOKBOOK

Guilt-free and Delicious ActiFry Recipe Ideas: Discover The Healthier Way to Fry!

Paperback / eBook

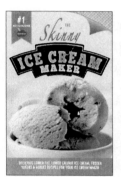

THE SKINNY ICE CREAM MAKER

Delicious Lower Fat, Lower Calorie Ice Cream, Frozen Yogurt & Sorbet Recipes For Your Ice Cream Maker.

Paperback / eBook

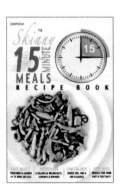

THE SKINNY 15 MINUTE MEALS RECIPE BOOK

Delicious, Nutritious & Super-Fast Meals in 15 Minutes Or Less. All Under 300, 400 & 500 Calories.

Paperback / eBook

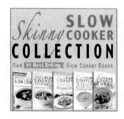

THE SKINNY SLOW COOKER COLLECTION

5 Fantastic Books of Delicious, Diet-friendly Skinny Slow Cooker Recipes: ALL Under 200, 300, 400 & 500 Calories!
eBook

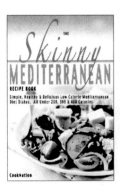

THE SKINNY MEDITERRANEAN RECIPE BOOK

Simple, Healthy & Delicious Low Calorie Mediterranean Diet Dishes. All Under 200, 300 & 400 Calories.

Paperback / eBook

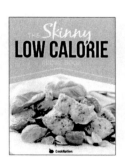

THE SKINNY LOW CALORIE RECIPE BOOK

Great Tasting, Simple & Healthy Meals Under 300, 400 & 500 Calories. Perfect For Any Calorie Controlled Diet.

Paperback / eBook

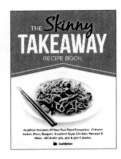

THE SKINNY TAKEAWAY RECIPE BOOK

Healthier Versions Of Your Fast Food Favourites: All Under 300, 400 & 500 Calories.

Paperback / eBook

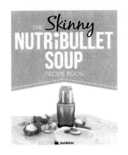

THE SKINNY NUTRIBULLET SOUP RECIPE BOOK

Delicious, Quick & Easy, Single Serving Soups & Pasta Sauces For Your Nutribullet. All Under 100, 200, 300 & 400 Calories!

Paperback / eBook

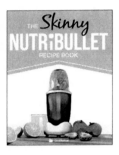

THE SKINNY NUTRIBULLET RECIPE BOOK

80+ Delicious & Nutritious Healthy Smoothie Recipes. Burn Fat, Lose Weight and Feel Great!

Paperback / eBook

CONVERSION CHART: DRY INGREDIENTS

Metric	Imperial
7g	¼ oz
15g	½ oz
20g	¾ oz
25g	1 oz
40g	1½oz
50g	2oz
60g	2½oz
75g	3oz
100g	3½oz
125g	4oz
140g	4½oz
150g	5oz
165g	5½oz
175g	6oz
200g	7oz
225g	8oz
250g	9oz
275g	10oz
300g	11oz
350g	12oz
375g	13oz
400g	14oz

Metric	Imperial
425g	15oz
450g	1lb
500g	1lb 2oz
550g	1¼lb
600g	1lb 5oz
650g	1lb 7oz
675g	1½lb
700g	1lb 9oz
750g	1lb 11oz
800g	1¾lb
900g	2lb
1kg	2¼lb
1.1kg	2½lb
1.25kg	2¾lb
1.35kg	3lb
1.5kg	3lb 6oz
1.8kg	4lb
2kg	4½lb
2.25kg	5lb
2.5kg	5½lb
2.75kg	6lb

CONVERSION CHART: LIQUID MEASURES

Metric	Imperial	US
25ml	1fl oz	
60ml	2fl oz	¼ cup
75ml	2½ fl oz	
100ml	3½fl oz	
120ml	4fl oz	½ cup
150ml	5fl oz	
175ml	6fl oz	
200ml	7fl oz	
250ml	8½ fl oz	1 cup
300ml	10½ fl oz	
360ml	12½ fl oz	
400ml	14fl oz	
450ml	15½ fl oz	
600ml	1 pint	
750ml	1¼ pint	3 cups
1 litre	1½ pints	4 cups

CPSIA information can be obtained at www.ICGtesting.com
Printed in the USA
BVOW03s1045080316

439351BV00069B/326/P